MATH NOTEBOOK

Everything you should know from

Kindergarten through Trigonometry

By: Leslie Schnorenberg

Note from the Author

Dear Students and Teachers,

I cannot tell you how excited I am to put this notebook in your hands as a tool you can use in your education and learning!

First, a note to the students: This notebook is designed as a tool for you to use as you progress through your Math studies from the most basic Math concepts to more challenging, complex concepts. I would encourage you to take the time to fill in the definitions and complete the examples for each page as you learn the importance of each concept in order to use the information as a reference and reminder of all you should know and understand in your Math studies from Kindergarten through Trigonometry.

This notebook will then become a perfect tool for any type of Math "test prep" as it will be extremely easy for you to go back and review all the key concepts you have learned up to your specific grade level!

Second, a note to the teachers: This notebook is designed to be a tool for you to use with your students to help them realize the important key concepts they should remember through their Math studies. This notebook is designed to keep Math simple and straightforward. Although it is not designed as a core curriculum, it is intended to streamline concepts and categorize learning in such a way that students are more apt to remember what they have learned and connect one idea to the next.

The checklist at the end of the book is also a tool designed to help identify where a student might have missed a key concept in their previous math studies. The checklist is "block building" in order to help students understand where they are in terms of their studies, and where they should be in order to complete the concepts needed for each level of Mathematics.

I welcome feedback of any kind for this resource. It is my hope and desire that in creating useful tools, our students will be given further help to succeed. Our nation is in serious need of a Math Revolution! We need students who understand and enjoy the study of Math. May this tool be useful toward such a goal!

Sincerely,

Leslie Schnorenberg

Table of Contents

- **Essentials of Elementary:**
  - Adding Natural Numbers (Carrying) 5
  - Subtracting Natural Numbers (Borrowing) 6
  - Multiplying Natural Numbers 7
  - Dividing Numbers 8
  - Kinds of Numbers 9
  - Place Values 10
  - Number Sets 11
- **Important Concepts of Pre-Algebra:**
  - Understanding Fractions 12
  - Understanding Mixed Numbers 13
  - Understanding Decimals 14
  - Understanding Percents 15
  - Factoring and Prime Factorization 16
  - Scientific Notation 17
  - Unit Conversions 18
  - Order of Operations 19
- **Important Concepts of Algebra:**
  - Integers 20
  - Variables and Numbers 21
  - Solving Algebraic Equations 22
  - Polynomials 23
  - Factoring Polynomials 24
  - Basics of Graphing 25
  - Linear Equations 26
  - Linear Inequalities 31
  - Matrices 33
  - Solving Systems of Equations 34
- **Important Concepts of Geometry:**
  - Points, Lines, and Planes 35
  - Angles 36
  - Names of Shapes 37
  - Triangles 38
  - Types of Quadrilaterals 41
  - Polygons: Area and Perimeter 42
  - Constructions 43
  - Circles 45
  - Hyperbolas 46
  - Ellipses 47
  - Polyhedrons 48
  - Transformations 49

    Translations 50
    Dilations 51
    Reflections 53
    Rotations 54
    Logic Statements 55
    Geometric Theorems and Postulates 57

❖ **Important Concepts of Advanced Algebra:**
    Complex Story Problems 60
    Functions 61
    Absolute Value Equations 62
    Powers and Roots 64
    Imaginary and Complex Numbers 65
    Quadratic Equations 66
    Polynomial Equations 69
    Inverse Functions 72
    Composite Functions 72
    Piece-Wise Functions 74
    Rational Functions 76
    Properties of Exponents 78
    Exponential Functions 79
    Properties of Logarithms 81
    Logarithmic Functions 82
    Arithmetic Sequences 84
    Geometric Sequences 85
    Combinations and Permutations 86

❖ **Basic Concepts of Statistics:**
    Statistic Basics 87
    Mean / Median / Mode 87
    Histogram / Bar Graph 87
    Box and Whisker Plots 87
    Bell Curves 87
    Standard Deviations 87
    Z-scores 87

❖ **Basic Concepts of Trigonometry:**
    Trigonometric Basics-Unit Circle 88
    Special Right Triangles 88
    Degrees and Radians 88
    Trigonometric Ratios 88

❖ **Math Mastery Checklist:**
    Checklist of Math Concepts 90

ADDING

What is an Addend and Sum:	Example: 3 + 8 =
What does it mean to add and what words are associated with "adding":	Example: 143 + 678 =
How do you add multiple digit numbers (carrying):	Example: 1,394 + 356
Properties of Addition: Commutative Property: Associative Property: Additive Identity Property:	Examples:

Fill out the Addition Table below:

1 + 1 =	1 + 2 =	1 + 3 =	1 + 4 =	1 + 5 =	1 + 6 =	1 + 7 =	1 + 8 =	1 + 9 =	1 + 10 =
2 + 1 =	2 + 2 =	2 + 3 =	2 + 4 =	2 + 5 =	2 + 6 =	2 + 7 =	2 + 8 =	2 + 9 =	2 + 10 =
3 + 1 =	3 + 2 =	3 + 3 =	3 + 4 =	3 + 5 =	3 + 6 =	3 + 7 =	3 + 8 =	3 + 9 =	3 + 10 =
4 + 1 =	4 + 2 =	4 + 3 =	4 + 4 =	4 + 5 =	4 + 6 =	4 + 7 =	4 + 8 =	4 + 9 =	4 + 10 =
5 + 1 =	5 + 2 =	5 + 3 =	5 + 4 =	5 + 5 =	5 + 6 =	5 + 7 =	5 + 8 =	5 + 9 =	5 + 10 =
6 + 1 =	6 + 2 =	6 + 3 =	6 + 4 =	6 + 5 =	6 + 6 =	6 + 7 =	6 + 8 =	6 + 9 =	6 + 10 =
7 + 1 =	7 + 2 =	7 + 3 =	7 + 4 =	7 + 5 =	7 + 6 =	7 + 7 =	7 + 8 =	7 + 9 =	7 + 10 =
8 + 1 =	8 + 2 =	8 + 3 =	8 + 4 =	8 + 5 =	8 + 6 =	8 + 7 =	8 + 8 =	8 + 9 =	8 + 10 =
9 + 1 =	9 + 2 =	9 + 3 =	9 + 4 =	9 + 5 =	9 + 6 =	9 + 7 =	9 + 8 =	9 + 9 =	9 + 10 =
10 + 1=	10 + 2=	10 + 3=	10 + 4=	10 + 5=	10 + 6=	10 + 7=	10 + 8=	10 + 9=	10 +10=

SUBTRACTING

What is a Minuend, Subtrahend and Difference:	Example: 8 − 3 =
What does it mean to subtract and what words are associated with "subtracting":	Example: 10 − 7 =
How do you subtract multiple digit numbers (borrowing):	Example: 1253 − 976

Fill out the Subtraction Table below:

1 - 1 =									
2 - 1 =	2 - 2 =								
3 - 1 =	3 - 2 =	3 - 3 =							
4 - 1 =	4 - 2 =	4 - 3 =	4 - 4 =						
5 - 1 =	5 - 2 =	5 - 3 =	5 - 4 =	5 - 5 =					
6 - 1 =	6 - 2 =	6 - 3 =	6 - 4 =	6 - 5 =	6 - 6 =				
7 - 1 =	7 - 2 =	7 - 3 =	7 - 4 =	7 - 5 =	7 - 6 =	7 - 7 =			
8 - 1 =	8 - 2 =	8 - 3 =	8 - 4 =	8 - 5 =	8 - 6 =	8 - 7 =	8 - 8 =		
9 - 1 =	9 - 2 =	9 - 3 =	9 - 4 =	9 - 5 =	9 - 6 =	9 - 7 =	9 - 8 =	9 - 9 =	
10 - 1=	10 - 2=	10 - 3=	10 - 4=	10 - 5=	10 - 6=	10 - 7=	10 - 8=	10 - 9 =	10-10 =

MULTIPLYING

What is a Factor and Product:	Example: 2 × 5 =
What does it mean to multiply and what words are associated with "multiplying":	Example: 7 × 6 =
How do you multiply multiple digit numbers:	Example: 127 ×43
Properties of Multiplication: Commutative Property: Associative Property: Multiplicative Identity Property:	Examples:

Fill out the Multiplication Table below:

	1	2	3	4	5	6	7	8	9	10	11	12
1												
2												
3												
4												
5												
6												
7												
8												
9												
10												
11												
12												

DIVIDING

What is a Dividend, Divisor and Quotient:	Example: $42 \div 6 =$
How do you divide multiple digit dividends:	Example: Rewrite Using Long Division: $1446 \div 6 =$
How do you divide multiple digit divisors:	Example: Rewrite Using Long Division: $2880 \div 12 =$
How do you divide leaving the remainder in fraction form:	Example: Rewrite Using Long Division: $71 \div 6 =$
How do you divide leaving the remainder in decimal form:	Example: Rewrite Using Long Division: $92 \div 8 =$
Rules of Divisibility: When is a number divisible by 2: When is a number divisible by 3: When is a number divisible by 5: When is a number divisible by 10:	Example: Is 60 divisible by 2? Why: Is 60 divisible by 3? Why: Is 60 divisible by 5? Why: Is 60 divisible by 10? Why:

KINDS OF NUMBERS

Fill in the chart below with the Hierarchy of Numbers:

What is a Real Number:	Example:
What is a Irrational Number:	Example:
What is an Rational Number:	Example:
What is an Integer:	Example:
What is a Whole Number:	Example:
What is a Counting/Natural Number:	Example:

PLACE VALUE

Fill out the Place Value Table below:

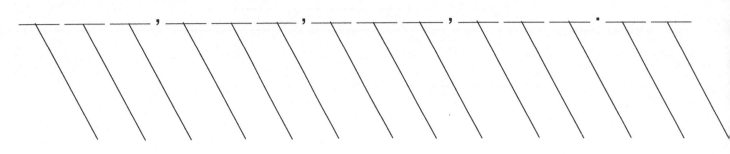

ROUNDING

What does it mean to round:	How do you round to a given place value: How do you determine if the number rounds up or down at that given place value:
How do you round to the nearest hundredths:	Example: Round the following number to the nearest hundredths: 134,532.576 ≈
How do you round to the nearest tens:	Example: Round the following numbers to the nearest tens: 134,532.576 ≈
How do you round to the nearest hundreds:	Example: Round the following numbers to the nearest hundred: 134,532.576 ≈
How do you round to the nearest ten thousands:	Example: Round the following numbers to the nearest ten thousands: 134,532.576 ≈

NUMBER SETS

What is a Number Set:	**Example:** $A = \{1,3,5,7,9\} \quad B = \{0,1,2,3,4\} \quad C = \{-1,2,4\}$
What is the Union of two sets? What symbol represents Union:	**Example:** Find $A \cup B =$
What is the Intersection of two sets? What symbol represents Intersection:	**Example:** Find $A \cap B =$
What is an Empty/Null Set? What symbol represents an Empty/Null Set:	**Example:** Find $A \cap C =$
What is a Venn Diagram:	**Example:** Create a Venn Diagram illustrating sets of numbers:

FRACTIONS

What is a Fraction? Which number is the Numerator? Which number is the Denominator:	**Example:** $$\frac{56}{8} =$$
How do you add/subtract Fractions with common denominators:	**Example:** $$\frac{2}{9} + \frac{4}{9} =$$
How do you add/subtract Fractions without common denominators (including Least Common Multiples):	**Example:** $$\frac{7}{9} + \frac{5}{12} =$$
How do you multiply Fractions:	**Example:** $$\frac{7}{8} \times \frac{16}{42} =$$
How do you divide Fractions:	**Example:** $$\frac{12}{16} \div \frac{3}{4} =$$
How do you change a Proper Fraction into an Improper Fraction and an Improper Fraction into a Proper Fraction:	**Example:** $$1\frac{4}{9} =$$ $$\frac{39}{9} =$$
How do you simplify Fractions (including Greatest Common Factor):	**Example:** $$\frac{88}{16} =$$

MIXED NUMBERS

What is a Mixed Number?	Example: Give an example of a Mixed Number:
How do you add Mixed Numbers:	Example: $4\dfrac{2}{9} + 8\dfrac{1}{3} =$
How do you subtract Mixed Numbers:	Example: $10\dfrac{3}{8} - 6\dfrac{5}{12} =$
How do you multiply Mixed Numbers:	Example: $5\dfrac{1}{2} \times 6\dfrac{3}{4} =$
How do you divide Mixed Numbers:	Example: $4\dfrac{1}{2} \div 2\dfrac{1}{4} =$

DECIMALS

What is a Decimal:	**Example:** .0876
How do you add/subtract Decimals:	**Example:** .0937 + 2.468
How do you multiply Decimals:	**Example:** .093 ×2.46
How do you divide Decimals with a Decimal as the Dividend:	**Example:** Rewrite using Long Division: $1.69 \div 13 =$
How do you divide Decimals with a Decimal as the Divisor:	**Example:** Rewrite using Long Division: $2.25 \div .15 =$
How do you change a Fraction into a Decimal:	**Example:** $\dfrac{39}{8} =$
How do you change a Decimal into a Fractions:	**Example:** .096 =

PERCENTS

What is a Percent:	Example: 97%
How do you convert a Percentage into a Decimal:	Example: 46% =
How do you convert a Percentage into a Fraction:	Example: 32% =
How do you find the Percentage of a number:	Example: What is 25% *of* $45.00 =
How do you answer story problems with Percentages:	Example: 24 students in a class took an algebra test. If 18 students passed the test, what percent do <u>not</u> pass?

FACTORING AND PRIME FACTORIZATION

What is a Composite Number:	**Example:** List the Composite Numbers from 0-20:
What is a Prime Number:	**Example:** List the Prime Numbers from 0-20:
How do you factor a Composite Number:	**Example:** Factor the following number: 45
What is the Prime Factorization of a Composite Number:	**Example:** Factor the following number with Prime Factorization: 540
How do you use Exponents in Prime Factorization:	**Example:** Factor the following number with Prime Factorization and Exponents: 540

SCIENTIFIC NOTATION

How do you put a number in Scientific Notation:	**Example:** $1{,}456{,}000 =$
How do you put a Whole Number in Scientific Notation:	**Example:** $2{,}300{,}000{,}000{,}000 =$
How do you put a Decimal Number in Scientific Notation:	**Example:** $.0002567 =$
How do you convert from Scientific Notation to Standard Notation with positive exponents:	**Example:** $2.987 \times 10^7 =$
How do you convert from Scientific Notation to Standard Notation with negative exponents:	**Example:** $2.987 \times 10^{-7} =$

UNIT CONVERSIONS

What are Metric Units of Measurement and what do they measure:	What are Customary Units of Measurement and what do they measure:
Meter:	Mile, Yard, Foot, Inch:
Liter:	Gallon, Quart, Pint, Cup:
Gram:	Ton, Pound, Ounce:

List the Order of Metric Prefixes in the Chart Below (use Meters as an Example):

1000   100   10   1 . 0.1   0.01   0.001   0.0001

How do you use the chart above to do Metric Unit Conversions:	Example: Convert 300 milligrams to kilograms:
	Use Scientific Notation to Re-Write this:
What are the Unit Conversions for the Customary System:	**Example:** Convert 3 miles to inches:
1 Mile = _____ Yards 1 Yard = _____ Feet 1 Foot = _____ Inches 1 Inch ≈ _____ Centimeters 1 Gallon = _____ Quarts 1 Quarts = _____ Pints 1 Pint = _____ Cups 1 Ton = _____ Pounds 1 Pound = _____ Ounces	Convert 10 cups to gallons:

ORDER OF OPERATIONS

What is the Order of Operations:	What is the saying to help with the Order of Operations:
What does PEMDAS stand for: P: E: M: D: A: S:	**Examples:** $18 \div 9 + 6 \times 3 - 5 =$ $\dfrac{6^2 - 2(3 + 10)}{5} =$ $\dfrac{2^3 - (2 - 10)}{2^2 + 4} =$
What is the Distributive Property:	**Example:** $3(4 + 6) =$ $3(4x + 6y) =$

INTEGERS

What is an Integer:	Examples:
How do you add Integers:	**Example:** $-3 + -6 =$ $-7 + 4 =$
How do you subtract Integers:	**Example:** $-3 - (-6) =$ $-7 - 4 =$
What are the rules for multiplying Integers:	**Example:** $-3 \cdot -6 =$ $-3 \cdot 6 =$ $3 \cdot -6 =$ $3 \cdot 6 =$
What are the rules for dividing Integers:	**Example:** $-12 \div -2 =$ $-12 \div 2 =$ $12 \div -2 =$ $12 \div 2 =$
What happens when you divide by zero:	**Example:** $2 \div 0 =$

VARIABLES AND NUMBERS

What is a Variable:	Example: $a, b, c, \ldots x, y, z$
What is a Co-efficient:	Example: $7x, -98y, 3x^3$
What is a Term:	Example: $7x, -98y, 3x^3$
What are Like Terms:	Example: $7x^2$ and $32x^2$; $-9a^{10}$ and $24a^{10}$
What is an Algebraic Expression:	Example: $7x^2 + 6xy$
What is an Algebraic Equation:	Example: $7 + 6x = 13$
How do you add/subtract Variables:	Example: $7x^2 + 9x^2y - 3x^2 + 4yx^2 =$
How do you multiply Variables:	Example: $7x^2 \cdot 6xy =$
How do you divide Variables:	Example: $\dfrac{14x^2}{42xy} =$

21

SOLVING ALGEBRAIC EQUATIONS

What does it mean to "solve an algebraic equation":	**Example:** $6x + 10 = 64$
How do you solve addition equations:	**Example:** $x + 12 = 35$
How do you solve subtraction equations:	**Example:** $x - 14 = 22$
How do you solve multiplication equations:	**Example:** $6x = 42$
How do you solve division equations:	**Example:** $\dfrac{x}{3} = 9$
How do you solve complex algebraic equations:	**Example:** $\dfrac{1}{3}(5x + 10) - 5 = 25$

POLYNOMIALS

What is a Polynomial:	Example: $6x^2 + 3x + 10$
How do you add Polynomials:	Example: $(6x^2 + 3x + 10) + (9x^2 + 7x - 2) =$
How do you subtract Polynomials:	Example: $(6x^2 + 3x + 10) - (9x^2 + 7x - 2) =$
How do you multiply Polynomials:	Example: $6xy(9x^2 + 7x - 2) =$
What is FOIL and how do you use it:	Example: $(3x + 5)(4x - 2) =$
How do you divide Polynomials:	Example: $\dfrac{(6xy^2 + 4xy + 10y)}{2y} =$ $\dfrac{(x^2 + 6x + 9)}{(x + 3)} =$

FACTORING POLYNOMIALS

How do you factor a term out of a Polynomial:	Example: $$12x^2y - 3xy - 6y =$$
How do you factor Polynomials with four terms:	Example: $$x^2 - 2x + 3x - 6 =$$
How do you factor Polynomials without an "a" term:	Example: $$x^2 - 5x - 6 =$$
How do you factor Polynomials with an "a" term:	Example: $$6x^2 - 17x + 12 =$$

GRAPHING

Which variable is the Independent Variable:	Which variable is the dependent Variable:
What is the Domain of a Function:	What is the Range of a Function:
What is a Cartesian Plane? **Where is the x-axis? Where is the y-axis?** **How do you plot points:** In each Quadrant, is x and y positive or negative: Quadrant I = (,) Quadrant II = (,) Quadrant III = (,) Quadrant IV = (,)	**Example:** Make an x and y axis Plot the points: $(-1,2); (3,5); (4,-3); (-5,-4)$ State the Domain and Range for the function above: Domain: Range:

25

LINEAR EQUATIONS

What are the three forms of a Linear Equation:

1)

2)

3)

What is Slope and what is its formula:	**Example:** Find the slope between the two points: $(1,2)$ and $(7,-9)$
What is a Table of Values:	**Example:** Create a Table of Values with three points for the function: $y = 4x - 3$
What information does the Standard Form of a Linear Equation tell you, and how do you graph with it:	**Example:** Graph: $2x + 3y = 12$

LINEAR EQUATIONS continued

What information does the Slope-Intercept Form of a Linear Equation tell you, and how do you graph with it:	**Example:** Graph $y = \frac{2}{3}x - 5$

What information does the Point-Slope form of a Linear Equation tell you, and how do you graph with it:	**Example:** Graph: $(y - 5) = 2(x + 1)$

LINEAR EQUATIONS continued

How do you find a Linear Equation given slope and a y-intercept:	**Example:** Find the equation of the line with slope $-1/2$ and y-intercept $(0, -6)$:
How do you find a Linear Equation given slope and a point:	**Example:** Find the equation of the line with slope 3 going through the point $(4, -5)$:
How do you find a Linear Equation given two points:	**Example:** Find the equation of the line going through the points $(2, -5)$ and $(5, 7)$:

LINEAR EQUATIONS continued

What is the relationship between two Parallel Lines:	**Example:** Write an equation for a line going through point (10,4) parallel to the line $y = -\frac{1}{5}x + 13$:
What do you know about their slopes:	
What is the relationship between two Perpendicular Lines:	**Example:** Write an equation for a line going through point (2,4) perpendicular to the line $y = -\frac{1}{5}x + 13$:
What do you know about their slopes:	

GRAPHS OF LINEAR EQUATIONS

Graph the following equations on the same axis to see what happens when numbers change:

1) $y = x$

2) $y = x + 3$

3) $y = 2x + 3$

4) $y = -2x + 3$

5) $y = -\dfrac{1}{2}x - 3$

6) $y = -5$

7) $x = -5$

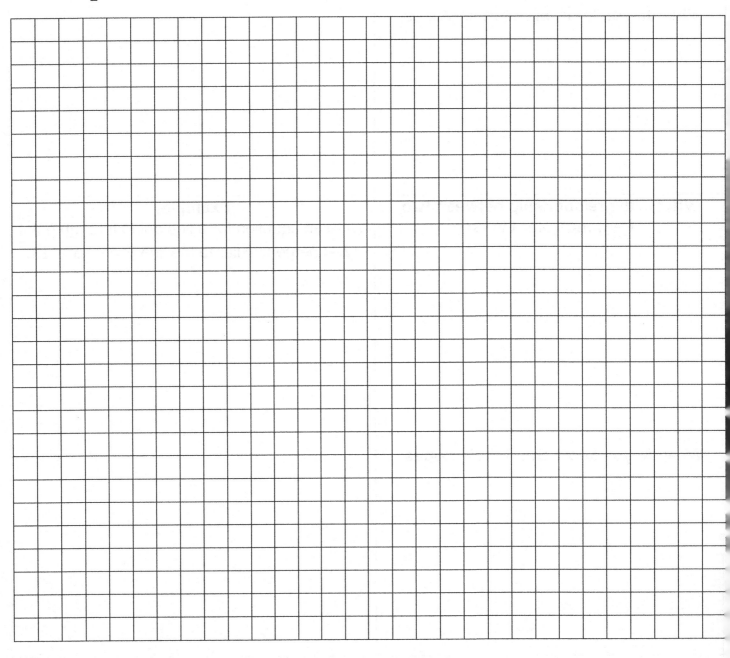

LINEAR INEQUALITIES:

What do the following symbols mean: $<$ $>$ $\leq$ $\geq$	How do you solve an Inequality? Solve the following Inequality: $-2x - 3 < 5$ *What is the one special rule you must remember when solving Inequalities?
How do you graph an Inequality on a number line? If the equation has either a < or > symbol, is the dot open or closed? Why: If the equation has either a $\leq$ or $\geq$ symbol, is the dot open or closed? Why:	Example: Solve each Inequality, then graph it on the number line: $-2x - 3 < 5$ ⟵—————————⟶ $-2x - 3 \geq 5$ ⟵—————————⟶
When graphing a Linear Inequality on a Cartesian plane containing either a $\leq$ or $\geq$, should the line be dotted or solid? Why:	When graphing a Linear Inequality on a Cartesian plane containing either a $<$ or $>$, should the line be dotted or solid? Why:
How do you determine which side of the dotted or solid line should be shaded?	If two Linear Inequalities are graphed on the same axis, how do you determine the solution set?

GRAPHS OF LINEAR INEQUALITIES

Graph the following inequalities on the same axis. Remember to check:

1) Dotted or Solid? 2) Which side is shaded? 3) If more than one inequality, what is the final solution set?

1) $y > -2$

2) $x < 5$

3) $y \geq x + 1$

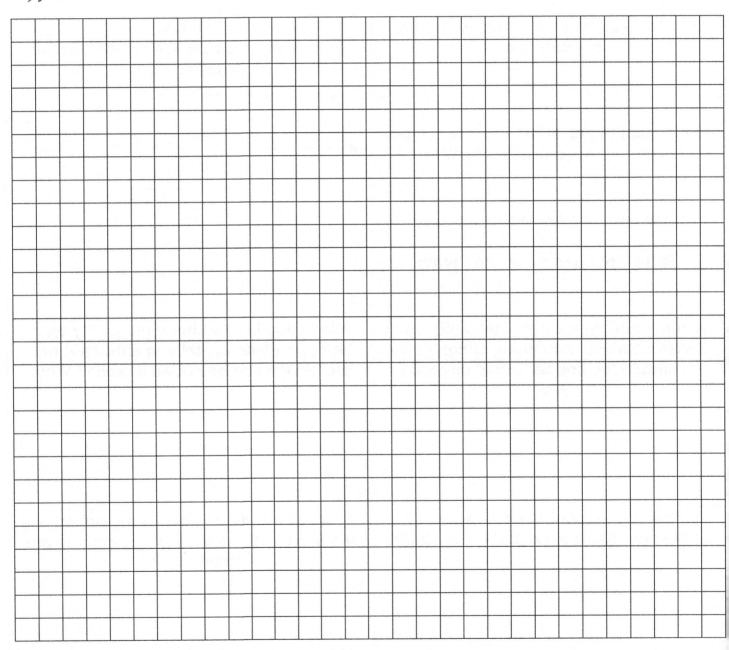

MATRICES

What is a Matrix?	**Example:** $$A = \begin{bmatrix} 2 & -4 \\ 3 & 5 \end{bmatrix}$$
How do you add Matrices:	**Example:** $$\begin{bmatrix} 2 & -4 \\ 3 & 5 \end{bmatrix} + \begin{bmatrix} 5 & -2 \\ -9 & 1 \end{bmatrix} =$$
How do you subtract Matrices:	**Example:** $$\begin{bmatrix} 2 & -4 \\ 3 & 5 \end{bmatrix} - \begin{bmatrix} 5 & -2 \\ -9 & 1 \end{bmatrix} =$$
How do you multiply Matrices:	**Example:** $$\begin{bmatrix} 2 & 1 & 4 \\ 6 & 0 & -1 \end{bmatrix} \cdot \begin{bmatrix} 4 & -5 \\ 3 & 10 \\ 2 & 7 \end{bmatrix} =$$
How do you find an Inverse Matrix:	**Example:** Find the inverse of the following matrix: $$\begin{bmatrix} 1 & 3 & 3 \\ 1 & 4 & 3 \\ 1 & 3 & 4 \end{bmatrix} =$$
What is a Matrix Identity:	**Example:** What is the 2x2 Identity Matrix?

SOLVING SYSTEMS OF EQUATIONS

How do you solve a System of Equations by Graphing:	**Example:** Graph: $y = 2x - 3$ $\quad 2x + 3y = -9$
How do you solving a System of Equations by Elimination:	**Example:** $8x - 6y = -6$ $2x + 3y = -9$
How do you solving a System of Equations by Substitution:	**Example:** $y = 4x - 7$ $2x + 3y = -9$
How do you solve a System of Equations using Matrices:	**Example:** $4x - 3y = -3$ $2x + 3y = -9$

POINTS, LINES, AND PLANES

What is the definition of a Point:	What is the definition of a Segment:
What is the definition of a Ray:	**What is the definition of a Line:**
How do you find the distance between two points on a Line: (Distance Formula):	**Example:** Find the distance between the two points: (2,6) and (6,9):
How do you find the midpoint between two points on a Line: (Midpoint Formula):	**Example:** Find the midpoint between the two points: (2,6) and (6,12): Find the endpoint if one endpoint is at (2,6) and the midpoint is at (6,12):

ANGLES

What is the definition of an Angle:	What are the three ways to name an Angle:
What are the classifications of an Angle? Define each and draw an example of each: Acute: Right: Obtuse: Straight:	**What are the different types of Angles? Define each and draw and example of each:** Vertical: Alternate Interior: Alternate Exterior: Corresponding: Adjacent: Complimentary: Supplementary:

NAMES OF SHAPES

What does it mean when a shape is Concave:	**What does it mean when a shape is Convex:**
Draw and define a Triangle:	**Draw and define a Quadrilateral:**
Draw and define a Pentagon:	**Draw and define a Hexagon:**
Draw and define a Heptagon:	**Draw and define an Octagon:**
Draw and define a Nonagon:	**Draw and define a Decagon:**
Draw and define a Dodecagon:	**Draw and define an Icosagon:**
What does it mean that a shape is "Regular":	**Just for fun: How many sides does a Tetracontakaihexagon have?**

TRIANGLES

What are the classifications of Triangles by their Angle Measures? Define each and draw an example:	What are the classifications of Triangles by their Side Lengths? Define each and draw an example:
Acute:	**Equilateral:**
Right:	**Isosceles:**
Obtuse:	**Scalene:**

What is the Triangle Sum Theorem:	**Example:** Find the missing angle measure if $\angle A = 47°$ and $\angle B = 71°$:

What is the Triangle Inequality Theorem and what does it tell you about the length of a third side, if given the measurements of the other two sides:	**Example:** What is the minimum and maximum length the third side of a triangle can be, if two sides of the triangle are 5in and 7in.?

What are the properties of Congruent Triangles? Explain each of the following:	**What are the properties of Similar Triangles? Explain each of the following:**
SSS	SSS~
SAS	
ASA	AA~
AAS	SAS~
HL	

TRIANGLES continued

What is the Pythagorean Theorem and how to do you use it to find the missing side measure of a right triangle?	**Example:** Find the missing side measure of a right triangle if the hypotenuse is 15 and a leg measure is 9.
What is the Pythagorean Inequality Theorem and how does it tell you if the triangle is acute or obtuse?	**Example:** Using the Pythagorean Inequality Theorem, tell whether the following triangles are obtuse or acute: 3-4-6: 10-14-16:
What is the Exterior Angle Inequality?	**Example:** Fill in the inequality below: $\angle ABC$ _____ $\angle BCD$
What is the relationship between triangle angles and their opposite sides?	**Example:** Label the angles below smallest to largest: (triangle with sides 15, 6, 8)

39

TRIANGLES continued

What are the formulas for Special Right Triangles and how do you use them to find missing side measures: 45-45-90: 30-60-90:	**Example:** Find the missing side measure of the following triangles: 2 9
What are the three basic Trigonometric Ratios: Sine: Cosine: Tangent: What saying helps you remember these ratios:	**What are their Reciprocal Ratios:** Cosecant: Secant: Cotangent:
How do you use the Trigonometric Ratios to find missing side measures:	**How do you use the Trigonometric Ratios to find missing angle measures:**

TYPES OF QUADRILATERALS

Fill in the chart below with the Hierarchy of Quadrilaterals:

What is a Quadrilateral? Draw an example and list its properties:	What is a Parallelogram? Draw an example and list its properties:
What is a Rectangle? Draw an example and list its properties:	**What is a Rhombus? Draw an example and list its properties:**
What is a Square? Draw an example and list its properties:	**What is a Trapezoid? Draw an example and list its properties:**
What is a Kite? Draw an example and list its properties:	**Example Question:** Are all rhombuses parallelograms? Are all parallelograms rhombuses?

AREA AND PERIMETER

What is perimeter:	What is area:
What is the formula for the perimeter of a Triangle:	What is the formula for the area of a Triangle:
What is the formula for the perimeter of a Rhombus:	What is formula for the area of a Rhombus:
What is the formula for the perimeter of a Square:	What is the formula for the area of a Square:
What is the formula for the perimeter of a Rectangle/Parallelogram:	What is the formula for the area of a Rectangle/Parallelogram:
What is the formula for the perimeter of a Trapezoid:	What is the formula for the area of a Trapezoid:
What is the formula for the perimeter of a N-gon:	What is the formula for the area of a N-gon:
What is the formula for degree measure of Exterior Angles:	What is the formula for the sum of the degree measure of Interior Angles:

CONSTRUCTIONS:

What is a Geometric Construction:	What are the only tools you can use when Constructing:
How do you Construct a Segment congruent to the given Segment:	**Example:** Construct a Segment congruent to the given Segment: _____
How do you Construct a Perpendicular Bisector:	**Example:** Construct the Perpendicular Bisector of the Segment below: _____
How do you Construct a line perpendicular to a given line through a given point:	**Example:** Construct a line perpendicular to the given line through the given point: • _____
How do you Construct an angle congruent to the given angle:	**Example:** Construct an angle congruent to the given angle:

CONSTRUCTIONS AND TRIANGLES:

What is an Angle Bisector and how do you construct it:	**Example:** Construct an Angle Bisector to the given angle:
What is a Triangle's Incenter and how do you find it: **What is an Angle Bisector:**	**Example:** Construct the Incenter finding each Angle Bisectors:
What is a Triangle's Circumcenter, and how do you find it: **What is a Perpendicular Bisector:**	**Example:** Construct the Circumcenter by finding the perpendicular bisectors:
What is a Triangle's Centroid, and how do you find it: **What is a Median:**	**Example:** Construct the Centroid by finding the medians:
What is a Triangle's Orthocenter, and how do you find it: **What is an Altitude:**	**Example:** Construct the Orthocenter by finding the altitudes:

CIRCLES

What are the parts of a Circle? Define each:	How do you find Arc Measures? Give the formula for each:
Radius:	Circumference Formula:
Diameter:	
Circumference:	Central Arc Measure:
Chord:	
Tangent Line:	Arcs of Inscribed Angles:
Secant Line:	
Major Arc:	Arcs of Intersecting Secant and Tangent Lines:
Minor Arc:	
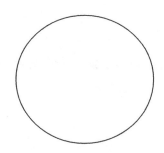	Arcs of Intersecting Secant Lines:
How do you find the area of a Sector:	What is the formula for a Circle, and how do you graph it:
Area Formula:	Circle Formula:
Sector Formula:	

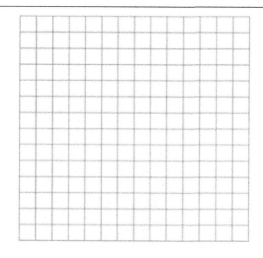

Graph the following Circle Equations to see how the numbers change the graph:

1) $x^2 + y^2 = 9$

2) $x^2 + y^2 = 16$

3) $(x-2)^2 + (y+3)^2 = 9$

HYPERBOLAS

How do you graph a Hyperbola:	How do find the center of a Hyperbola:
Hyperbola Formula: **Vertical:** **Horizontal:**	 **How do you find the asymptotes of a Hyperbola:** **How do you find the foci of a Hyperbola:**

Graph the following Hyperbola Equations to see how the numbers change the graph:

1) $\dfrac{x^2}{9} - \dfrac{y^2}{16} = 1$

2) $\dfrac{(x-2)^2}{9} - \dfrac{(y+1)^2}{16} = 1$

3) $\dfrac{y^2}{9} - \dfrac{x^2}{16} = 1$

4) $\dfrac{(y-2)^2}{9} - \dfrac{(x+1)^2}{16} = 1$

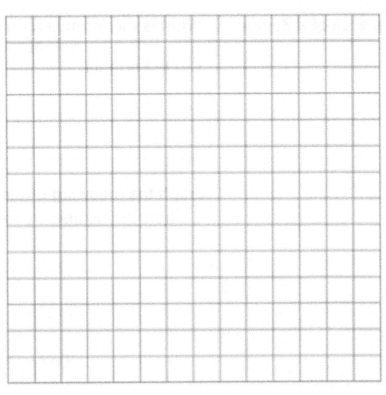

46

ELLIPSES

How do you graph an Ellipse:	How do find the center of an Ellipse:
Ellipse Formula:	
How do you determine the major axis:	**How do you find the foci of a Ellipse:**

Graph the following Ellipse Equations to see how the numbers change the graph:

1) $\dfrac{x^2}{9} + \dfrac{y^2}{16} = 1$

2) $\dfrac{(x-2)^2}{9} + \dfrac{(y+1)^2}{16} = 1$

3) $\dfrac{y^2}{9} + \dfrac{x^2}{16} = 1$

4) $\dfrac{(y-2)^2}{9} + \dfrac{(x+1)^2}{16} = 1$

POLYHEDRONS

What is a Polyhedron:	Pyramids:
	Volume:
	Surface Area:

Prisms:	Cones:
Volume:	Volume:
Surface Area:	Surface Area:

Cylinders:	Spheres:
Volume:	Volume:
Surface Area:	Surface Area:

TRANSFORMATIONS

What are the four types of Transformations? Give names and definitions for each:

1)

2)

3)

4)

What are the properties of Congruent Figures:

What are the properties of Similar Figures:

Ratios/Proportions of Similar Figures:

Perimeter:

Area:

Volume:

Examples:
What is the ratio of the Perimeter, Area and Volume of two similar figures if their scale factor is 3:5:

TRANSLATIONS

What is a Translation:	**Draw an Example:**

How do you identify corresponding parts of translated figures: **How do you label corresponding parts:**	**Example:** Identify the corresponding parts of the two figures below and label them: **Figure 1** **Figure 2**

How do you graph a translation:	**Example:** Graph the triangle: $A(0,0)$; $B(3,0)$; $C(3,5)$ under the translation: $(x+3, y-4)$ and label the figures:

50

DILATIONS: STRETCHING/SHRINKING

What is a Shrinking:	What is Shrinking:
What is a scale factor and how do you find it? If a scale factor is > than 1, then the image is: _____ If a scale factor is < than 1, then the image is: _____ (stretching or shrinking)	**Example:** Find the scale factor of the two images below: 3 7.5
Given the side measures, how do you determine if one figure is a dilation of the other?	**Example:** Determine if the two shapes are similar: 9, 15, 12 3, 5, 4
How do find the missing side measure of a dilation using proportions:	**How do you find the missing side measure of an dilation using scale factors:**
How do you graph a dilation:	**Example:** Graph the triangle: $(0,0); (3,0); (3,5)$ under the enlargement $(2x, 2y)$ and $(\frac{1}{2}x, \frac{1}{2}y)$:

DILATION: STRETCHING/SHRINKING

Subtopic: RATIOS & PROPORTIONS

What is a ratio and what are the two ways you can write a ratio:	What is a proportion:
How do you set up proportions: Which numbers are the means: Which numbers are the extremes:	**Example:** Write a proportion for the parts of the triangles below: [Triangle 1: legs 9 and Y, hypotenuse X] [Triangle 2: legs 3 and 4, hypotenuse 5]
How do you solve a proportion:	**Example:** Solve the following proportion: $$\frac{x}{100} = \frac{5}{25}$$
How do you solve story problems with proportions:	**Example:** At 3:00 in the afternoon, a building 90 feet tall cast a shadow 15 feet long. At the same time and in the same location, how long would the shadow be a man 6 feet tall?

REFLECTIONS

What is a Reflection:	**Draw an Example:**
How do you graph a Reflection: Across the x-axis: $(x,y) \rightarrow (\quad , \quad)$ Across the y-axis: $(x,y) \rightarrow (\quad , \quad)$ Across the origin: $(x,y) \rightarrow (\quad , \quad)$ *	**Example:** Graph the triangle: (0,0); (3,0); (3,5) reflected over the x-axis, the y-axis and the origin:
What is Symmetry:	**What is Reflection Symmetry? Draw an example:** **What is Rotational Symmetry? Draw an example**

ROTATIONS

What is a Rotation:	**Fill in the blank:**
	Positive rotations go _____
	Negative Rotations go _____
	(Clockwise or Counterclockwise)
How do you graph a Rotation: Under a 90° rotation about the origin, $(x, y) \rightarrow (\ ,\ )$ Under a 180° rotation about the origin, $(x, y) \rightarrow (\ ,\ )$ Under a 270° rotation about the origin, $(x, y) \rightarrow (\ ,\ )$	**Example:** Graph the following shape under a 90°, 180°, and 270° counterclockwise rotation: (0,1); (4,2); (7,6)
Are Rotations Similar Figures? Explain why:	**Rotation Notation:** R(_____ , _____)

LOGIC STATEMENTS

What is a Conditional Statement:	**Example:** If it snows tomorrow, then I don't have school.
Which part of a Conditional Statement is the Hypothesis:	**Example:** State the Hypothesis of the Conditional Statement:
Which part of a Conditional Statement is the Conclusion:	**Example:** State the Conclusion of the Conditional Statement:
What is a Converse Statement:	**Example:** State the Converse of the Conditional Statement:
What is an Inverse Statement:	**Example:** State the Inverse of the Conditional Statement:
What is a Contrapositive Statement:	**Example:** State the Contrapositive of the Conditional Statement:
What is a Bi-Conditional Statement:	**Example:** Rewrite the Conditional Statement as a Bi-Conditional Statement:
What is a Truth Value:	**Example:** What is the truth value of the conditional statement: What is the truth value of the converse: What is the truth value of the inverse: What is the truth value of the contrapositive:
What is a Counter Example:	**Example:** Find a Counterexample to the Conditional Statement:

LOGIC STATEMENTS continued

What do the following symbols mean: $p \to q$ $\sim p \to \sim q$ $q \to p$ $\sim q \to \sim p$	Which symbols represent each of the following: The Conditional Statement: The Converse Statement: The Inverse Statement: The Contrapositive Statement:
How do you write a conditional statement from a Venn Diagram:	**Example:** Write a conditional statement for the following Venn Diagram: Have an ID card / All Students / Sally
What is Inductive Reasoning:	**Example:**
What is Deductive Reasoning:	**Example:**

GEOMETRIC THEOREMS AND POSTULATES

What is a Theorem:	What is a Postulate:

List of Theorems and Postulates to use in Geometric Proofs:

Euclid's Postulates
- Two points determine a line segment.
- A line segment can be extended indefinitely along a line.
- A circle can be drawn with a center and any radius.
- All right angles are congruent.
- If two lines are cut by a transversal, and the interior angles on the same side of the transversal have a total measure of less than 180 degrees, then the lines will intersect on that side of the transversal.

Segments and Lines
- **Betweenness Theorem:** If C is between A and B and on AB, then AC + CB = AB.
    - If A, B, and C are distinct points and AC + CB = AB, then C lies on AB.
    - For any points A, B, and C, AC + CB $\geq$ AB.
- **Dimension Assumption:** Given a line in a plane, there exists a point in the plane not on that line. Given a plane in space, there exists a line or a point in space not on that plane.
- **Distance Assumption:** On a number line, there is a unique distance between two points.
    - If two points lie on a plane, the line containing them also lies on the plane.
    - Through three non-colinear points, there is exactly one plane.
    - If two different planes have a point in common, then their intersection is a line.
- **Line Intersection Theorem:** Two different lines intersect in at most one point.
- **Number Line Assumption:** Every line is a set of points that can be put into a one-to-one correspondence with real numbers, with any point on it corresponding to zero and any other point corresponding to one. This was once called the Ruler Postulate.
- **Parallel Lines Theorem:** In a coordinate plane, two non-vertical lines are parallel if they have the same slope.
- **Perpendicular Lines Theorem:** In a coordinate plane, two non-vertical lines are perpendicular if the product of their slopes is -1.
- **Perpendicular Bisector Theorem:** If a point is on the perpendicular bisector of a segment, then it is equidistant from the endpoints of the segment. (Also, the converse is true).
- **Segment Addition Postulate:** For any segment, the measure of the whole is equal to the sum of the measures of its non-overlapping parts.
- **Unique Line Assumption:** Through any two points, there is exactly one line.

Angles
- **Alternate Interior Angles Theorem:** If two parallel lines are intersected by a transversal, then the alternate interior angles are equal in measure. (Also, the converse is true.)
- **Alternate Exterior Angles Theorem:** If two parallel lines are intersected by a transversal, then the alternate exterior angles are equal in measure. (Also, the converse is true.)
- **Angle Addition Postulate:** For any angle, the measure of the whole is equal to the sum of the measures of its non-overlapping parts.
- **Angle Bisector Theorem:** If a point is on the bisector of an angle, then it is equidistant from the sides of the angle. (Also, the converse is true.)
- **Congruent Complements Theorem:** Two angles that are both complementary to a third angle are congruent.
- **Congruent Supplements Theorem:** Two angles that are both supplementary to a third angle are congruent.
- **Corresponding Angles Postulate:** If two parallel lines are intersected by a transversal, then the corresponding angles are equal in measure. (Also, the converse is true.)
- **Definition of Complementary Angles:** Two angles whose measures have a sum of 90 degrees.
- **Definition of Supplementary Angles:** Two angles whose measures have a sum of 180 degrees.
- **Definition of Vertical Angles:** Two angles formed by intersecting lines and facing in the opposite direction.
- **Linear Pair Theorem:** If two angles form a linear pair, then they are supplementary.
- **Right Angle Congruence Theorem:** All right angles are congruent.

GEOMETRIC THEOREMS AND POSTULATES continued

Angles continued
- **Same-side Interior Angles Theorem:** If two parallel lines are intersected by a transversal, then alternate exterior angles are supplementary. (Also, the converse is true.)
- **Vertical Angles Theorem:** Vertical angles are equal in measure.

Triangles
- **Angle-Angle (AA) Similarity Postulate:** If two angles of one triangle are equal in measure to two angles of another triangle, then the two triangles are similar.
- **Angle-Angle-Side (AAS) Congruence Theorem:** If two angles and a non-included side of one triangle are equal in measure to the corresponding angles and side of another triangle, then the triangles are congruent.
- **Angle-Side-Angle (ASA) Congruence Postulate:** If two angles and the included side of one triangle are congruent to two angles and the included side of another triangle, then the triangles are congruent.
- **CPCTC:** When the corresponding parts of triangles are all equal, the triangles are congruent. (Also, the converse is true.)
- **Definition of Midsegments:** The midsegments of a triangle are parallel to the side with which they don't intersect, and half the length of that side.
- **Equilateral Triangle Theorem:** The sides and angles of an equilateral triangle are equal.
- **Exterior Angle Theorem:** An exterior angle of a triangle is equal in measure to the sum of the measures of its two remote interior angles.
    - The measure of an exterior angle of a triangle is greater than that of either remote interior angle.
- **Hypotenuse-Leg (HL) Congruence Theorem:** If the hypotenuse and a leg of a right triangle are congruent to the hypotenuse and leg of another right triangle, then the triangles are congruent.
- **Isosceles Triangle Theorem:** If two sides of a triangle are equal in measure, then the angles opposite those sides are equal in measure. (Also, the converse is true.)
- **Pythagorean Theorem:** $a^2 + b^2 = c^2$, if c is the hypotenuse.
- **Right Triangle Theorem:** The acute angles of a right triangle are complementary.
    - The altitude to the hypotenuse of a right triangle forms two similar triangles that are also similar to the original triangle.
- **Sides and Opposite Angles Theorem:** When two angles of a triangle are equal, their opposite sides are equal, and vice versa.
    - When two angles of a triangle are unequal, their opposite sides are unequal, and vice versa.
    - When two sides of a triangle are unequal, the longer side is opposite the larger angle, and vice versa.
- **Side-Angle-Side (SAS) Congruence Postulate:** If two sides and the included angle of one triangle are equal in measure to the corresponding sides and angle of another triangle, then the triangles are congruent.
- **Side-Angle-Side (SAS) Similarity Postulate:** If two sides of one triangle are proportional to two sides of another triangle and their included angles are congruent, then the triangles are similar.
- **Side-Side-Side (SSS) Congruence Postulate:** If three sides of one triangle are equal in measure to the corresponding sides of another triangle, then the triangles are congruent.
- **Side-Side-Side (SSS) Similarity Postulate:** If the three sides of one triangle are proportional to the three corresponding sides of another triangle, then the triangles are similar.
- **Third Angles Theorem:** If two angles of one triangle are congruent to two angles of another triangle, then the third pair of angles are congruent.
- **Triangle Inequality Theorem:** The sum of the lengths of any two sides of a triangle is greater than the length of the third side.
- **Triangle Sum Theorem:** The sum of the measure of the angles of a triangle is 180 degrees.

Polygons
- **Central Angles of Polygons Theorem:** The central angles of a regular polygon are congruent.
- **Definition of an Apothem:** Each apothem of a regular polygon bisects the central angle whose rays intersect the polygon at the vertices of the side to which the apothem is drawn.
- **Polygon Exterior Angle Theorem:** The sum of the exterior angles of a polygon is 360 degrees.
- **Polygon Interior Angles Theorem:** The angle sum of any n-sided polygon is $180(n - 2)$ degrees.
- **Polygon Diagonals Theorem:** The number of diagonals of any n-sided polygon is $½(n(n - 3))$.
- **Radii of Polygons Theorem:** The radii of a regular polygon bisect the interior angles.

GEOMETRIC THEOREMS AND POSTULATES continued

Quadrilaterals
- **Consecutive Angles of Parallelograms Theorem:** The consecutive angles of a parallelogram are supplementary.
- **Definition of a Parallelogram:** A quadrilateral is a parallelogram if (1) it has one pair of sides that are both parallel and congruent, (2) both pairs of opposite sides are congruent, (3) Both pairs of opposite angles are congruent, or (4) Its diagonals bisect each other.
- **Diagonals of Parallelograms Theorem:** The diagonals of a parallelogram bisect each other.
- **Diagonals of a Rhombus Theorem:** The diagonals of a rhombus bisect its interior angles.
- **Diagonals of a Rectangle Theorem:** The diagonals of a rectangle are congruent.
- **Isosceles Trapezoid Congruency Theorem:** The base angles, legs, and diagonals of an isosceles trapezoid are congruent.
- **Median of a Trapezoid Theorem:** The median of a trapezoid is parallel to its bases and the average of their lengths.
- **Opposite Sides and Angles of Parallelograms Theorem:** Both pairs of opposite sides and opposite angles in a parallelogram are congruent.

Circles
- **Congruent Chords Theorem:** Congruent chords in the same circle are equidistant from the center.
  - Congruent chords in the same circle define (cut) congruent arcs.
- **Chord-Chord Product Theorem:** If two chords intersect in the interior of a circle, then the products of the lengths of the segments of the chords are equal.
- **Definition of a Tangent Line:** A tangent line is perpendicular to the radius whose endpoint is the point of tangency.
- **Diameters and Chords Theorem:** A diameter that bisects a chord is perpendicular to it.
- **Inscribed Angle Theorem:** The measure of an inscribed angle is half the measure of its intercepted arc.
- **Intersecting Chords Theorem:** When chords intersect in the same circle, the products of their segments are equal.
- **Intersecting Secant Lines theorem:** When two secant segments share the same exterior endpoint, the products of the secant segments and their external segments are equal.
- **Parallel Chords Theorem:** Parallel chords cut congruent arcs.
- **Perpendicular Bisector of a Chord Theorem:** The perpendicular bisector of a chord contains the center of the circle.
- **Radii of Circles Theorem:** The radii of a circle are congruent.
- **Secant-Secant Product Theorem:** The measure of an angle whose sides are contained in distinct secant lines and whose vertex is in the interior of a circle is equal to half the sum of the measures of its intercepted arcs.
  - The measure of an angle whose vertex lies outside a circle, whose sides, when extended, both intersect the circle, is equal to half the difference of the measures of its intercepted arcs.
- **Secant-Tangent Product Theorem:** When a tangent segment and a secant segment share an exterior endpoint, the square of the length of the tangent segment is equal to the product of the secant segment with its external segment.
- **Tangent Lines Theorem:** Tangent segments from the same exterior point are congruent.
- **Central Angle Measures Theorem:** The measure of a central angle is equal to the measure of the arc it intercepts.

Properties of Equality
- **Addition Property of Equality:** If the same number is added to equal numbers, then the sums are equal.
- **Distributive Property of Equality:** $a(b + c) = ab + bc$
- **Division Property of Equality:** If equal numbers are divided by the same number, then the quotients are equal.
- **Multiplication Property of Equality:** If equal numbers are multiplied by the same number, then the products are equal.
- **Reflexive Property of Equality:** A number is equal to itself.
- **Substitution Property of Equality:** If values are equal, then one value may be substituted for the other.
- **Subtraction Property of Equality:** If the same number is subtracted from equal numbers, then the differences are equal.
- **Symmetric Property of Equality:** If $a = b$, then $b = a$.
- **Transitive Property of Equality:** If $a = b$ and $b = c$, then $a = c$.

COMPLEX STORY PROBLEMS

What are Distance/Rate/Time Problems? How do you set them up to solve them:

Example:
Jose left the White House and drove toward the recycling plant at an average speed of 40 km/h. Rob left some time later driving in the same direction at an average speed of 48 km/h. After driving for five hours, Rob caught up with Jose. How long did Jose drive before Rob caught up?

	DISTANCE	RATE	TIME
ROB			
JOSE			

What are Work Problems? How do you set them up to solve them:

Example:
Shawna can pour a large concrete driveway in six hours. Dan can pour the same driveway in seven hours. Find how long it would take them if they worked together.

What are Mixture Problems? How do you set them up to solve them:

Example:
9 lbs. of mixed nuts containing 55% peanuts were mixed with 6 lbs. of another kind of mixed nuts that contain 40% peanuts. What percent of the new mixture is peanuts?

	AMOUNT	PERCENT	TOTAL
MIX 1			
MIX 2			
TOTAL			

FUNCTIONS

What is a Relation:	What is a Function:
What is the difference between a Relation and a Function:	How do you use the Vertical Line Test to determine if a Relation is a Function:
What is Function Notation:	**Example:** $f(x), g(x), h(x)$
How do you find the value of a function, given x:	**Example:** Given $f(x) = 5x + 3$, find $f(3)$:
How do you add/subtract functions:	**Example:** Given $f(x) = 5x + 3$ and $g(x) = -4x + 6$, find $f(x) - g(x)$:
How do you multiply functions:	**Example:** Given $f(x) = 5x + 3$ and $g(x) = -4x + 6$, find $f(x) \cdot g(x)$:
How do you divide functions:	**Example:** Given $f(x) = 5x^3$ and $g(x) = 15x$, find $f(x) \div g(x)$:

ABSOLUTE VALUE EQUATIONS

What is an Absolute Value, and what shape is its graph:	Example: $$y = 3|x + 2| + 5$$
What is the basic Absolute Value Equation: **What do the values of a, h, and k do to the graph:** a: h: k:	Example: $$y = 3|x - 2| + 5$$
What is the Vertex and how do you find it:	Example: Find the vertex to the equation: $$y = 3|x + 2| + 5$$
How do you find the x-intercepts:	Example: Find the x-intercepts to the equation: $$y = -3|x + 2| + 5$$
How do you find the y-intercepts:	Example: Find the y-intercept to the equation: $$y = -3|x + 2| + 6$$
How do you solve an absolute value equation:	Example: Solve the following equation: $$17 = 3|x + 2| + 5$$

GRAPHS OF ABSOLUTE VALUE EQUATIONS

Graph the following equations on the same axis to see what happens when numbers change:

1) $y = |x|$

2) $y = |x + 3|$

3) $y = |x + 3| + 4$

4) $y = 2|x + 3| + 4$

5) $y = -\dfrac{1}{2}|x + 3| + 4$

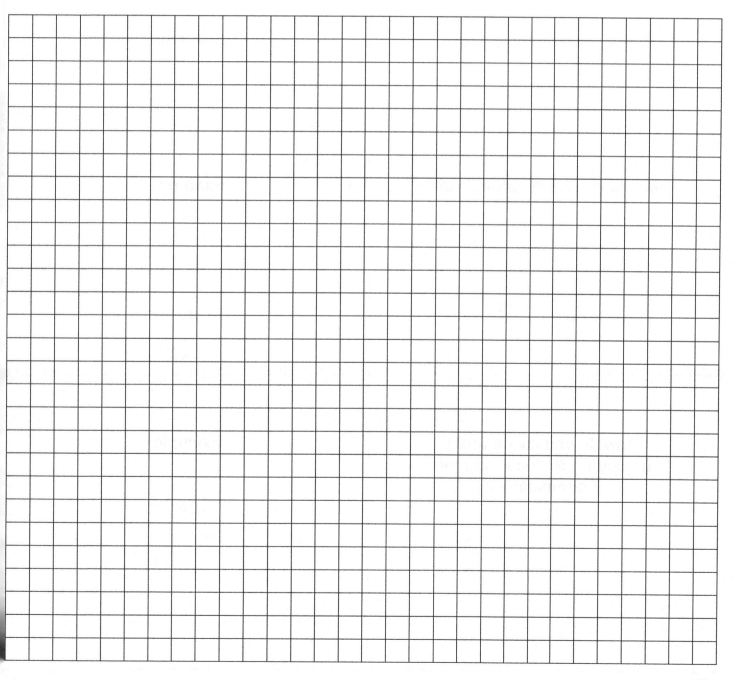

63

POWERS AND ROOTS

What is a Power (including squares and cubes):	Example: $8^2 =$ $3^3 =$
What is a Root (including square roots and cube roots):	Example: $\sqrt{36} =$ $\sqrt[3]{27} =$ $\sqrt[5]{243} =$
How do you simplify a root:	Example: $\sqrt{125} =$
How do you add/subtract roots:	Example: $\sqrt{8} + \sqrt{18} - \sqrt{2} =$
How do you multiply roots:	Example: $\sqrt{20} \cdot \sqrt{63} =$
How do you divide roots (including Rationalizing the Denominator):	Example: $\dfrac{\sqrt{63}}{\sqrt{18}} =$

IMAGINARY AND COMPLEX NUMBERS

What is an Imaginary Number:	**Example:**
What does the value *i* equal:	**Example:** Simplify the following Square Root values using i: $\sqrt{-2} =$ $\sqrt{-4} =$ $\sqrt{-6} =$
How do the following *i* values simplify: $i =$ $i^2 =$ $i^3 =$ $i^4 =$	**Example:** Simplify the values of the following i values: $i^{99} =$ $i^{24} =$
What is a Complex Number, and what form is it written in:	**Example:** $8 - 2i$
What is a Complex Conjugate:	**Example:** Find the Complex Conjugate of the following: $8 - 2i$
How do you use Complex Conjugates to simplify Complex Rational Numbers:	**Example:** $\dfrac{8 - 2i}{6 + 3i} =$

QUADRATIC EQUATIONS

What is a Quadratic Equation, and what shape is its graph:	**Example:** $y = 3x^2 + 7x + 10$ $y = (x+7)(x+10)$ $y = 3(x+7)^2 + 10$
What is the Standard form for a Quadratic Equation:	**Example:** $y = 3x^2 + 7x + 10$
What is the Vertex form of a Quadratic Equation: **What do the values of a, h, and k do to the graph:** a: h: k:	**Example:** $y = 3(x+7)^2 + 10$
How do you determine if the graph opens up or down?	**Example:** Tell whether the graph opens up or down: $y = -3x^2 + 7x + 10$ $y = 3x^2 + 7x + 10$
What is a y-intercept? How do you find it:	**Example:** Find the y-intercept for the following equation: $y = x^2 + 7x + 10$
What is the Discriminant? **If the Discriminant=0, what does that tell you about the graph?** **If the Discriminant>0, what does that tell you about the graph?** **If the Discriminant<0, what does that tell you about the graph?**	**Example:** Find the Discriminant and determine what it tells you about the graph of the equation: $0 = x^2 + 7x + 10$

QUADRATIC EQUATIONS continued

What is an x-intercept? How do you find them:	Example:
1) Factoring 2) Completing the Square 3) Quadratic Formula	1) Solve by Factoring: $$0 = x^2 + 7x + 10$$ 2) Solve by Completing the Square: $$0 = x^2 + 7x + 10$$ 3) Solve by the Quadratic Formula: $$0 = x^2 + 7x + 10$$
What is the Vertex? What are the two methods for finding the Vertex: 1) 2)	Example: Find the vertex of the equation: $$y = x^2 + 7x + 10$$ Find the vertex of the equation: $$y = 3(x + 7)^2 + 2$$

GRAPHS OF QUADRATIC EQUATIONS

Graph the following equations on the same axis to see what happens when numbers change:

1) $y = x^2$

2) $y = (x+3)^2$

3) $y = (x+3)^2 + 4$

4) $y = 2(x-3)^2 + 4$

5) $y = -2(x-3)^2 + 4$

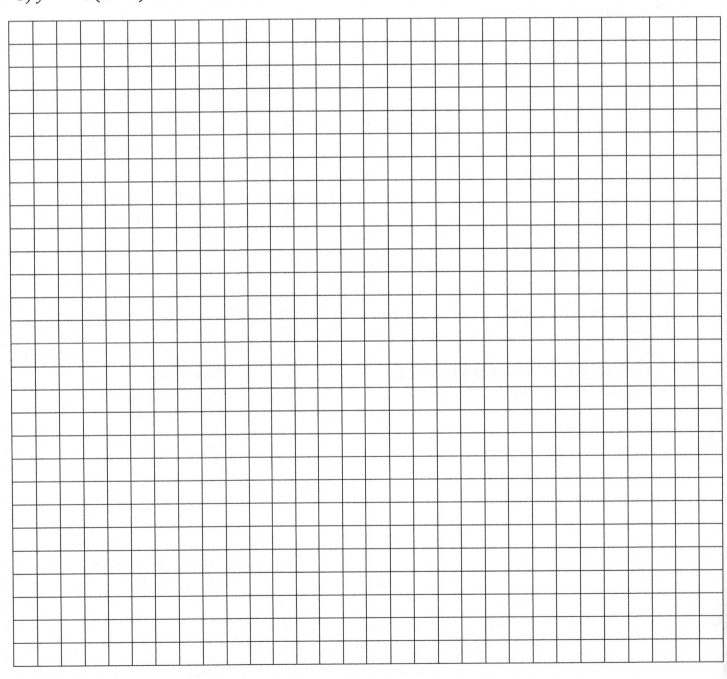

POLYNOMIAL EQUATIONS

What is a Polynomial Equation and how do you determine its degree:	Example: $$y = x^3 - 7x^2 + 16x - 10$$ $$y = 2(x-2)(x-4)^2(x+1)^2$$
What is the basic shape of an even degree polynomial function:	What is the basic shape of an odd degree polynomial function:
How do you determine the number of potential zeros in a polynomial function:	Example: Tell whether the function has an even or odd degree and how many potential zeros it has: $$y = 2(x-2)(x-4)^2(x+1)^2$$
How do you determine how many positive real roots the polynomial function has:	How do you determine how many negative real roots the polynomial function has:

What are the three methods you can use to find the roots/zeros of a polynomial function:

1)

2)

3)

POLYNOMIAL EQUATIONS continued

How do you factor a polynomial to find its roots:	**Example:** Find the roots of the polynomial using factoring: $$y = x^4 - 3x^2 + 2$$
How do you use long division to find a polynomial's roots:	**Example:** Find the roots of the polynomial using long division: $$y = 2x^3 + 9x^2 + 7x - 6,$$ if you know that $x = -3$ is one of the roots:
How do you use synthetic division to find a polynomial's roots:	**Example:** Find the roots of the polynomial using synthetic division: $$y = 2x^3 + 9x^2 + 7x - 6,$$ if you know that $x = -3$ is one of the roots:
What is the Synthetic Remainder Theorem:	**Example:** Using synthetic division, find the value of y when x=3: $$y = 2x^3 + 9x^2 + 7x - 6$$

GRAPHS OF POLYNOMIAL EQUATIONS

Graph the following equations on the same axis to see what happens when numbers change:

1) $y = 2x^3 + 9x^2 + 7x - 6$ $\qquad\qquad y = 2(x-2)(x-4)^2(x+1)^2$

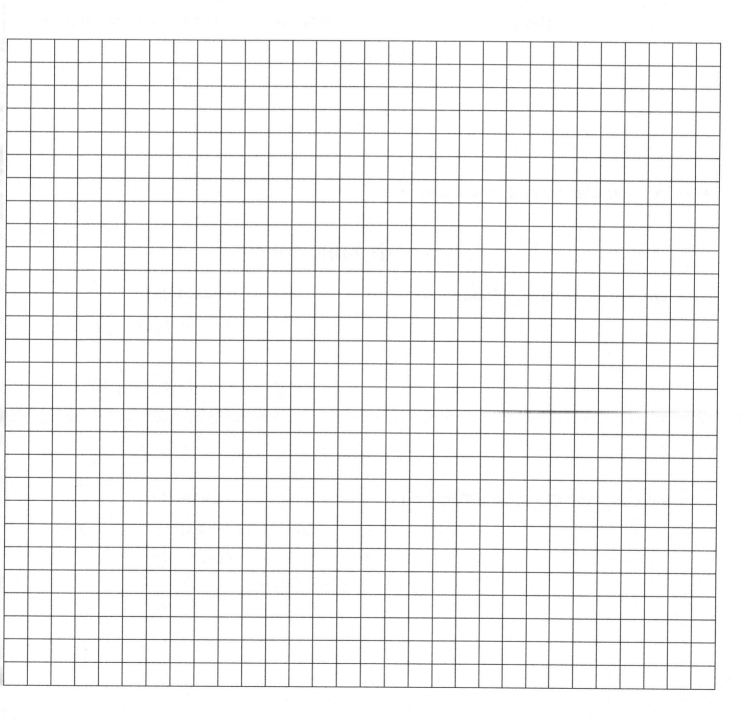

INVERSE EQUATIONS

What are Inverse Functions:	Example: $$y = \frac{1}{2}x + 9$$ and $$y = 2(x - 9)$$
How do you find the Inverse of a function:	Example: Find the inverse of the following function: $$y = \frac{1}{3}x - 7$$
How do their domain and range compare:	

COMPOSITE FUNCTIONS

What are Composite Functions:	Example: $$g(x) = 2x + 9 \text{ and } f(x) = \frac{1}{3}x + 10$$ $$g(f(x)) = 2\left(\frac{1}{3}x + 10\right) + 9$$ $$= \frac{2}{3}x + 29$$
How do you find Composite Functions:	Example: $$g(x) = 2x + 9 \text{ and } f(x) = \frac{1}{3}x + 10$$ Find $f(g(x))$:

GRAPHS OF INVERSE EQUATIONS

Graph the following equations on the same axis to see what happens:

1) $y = 3x + 4$

2) $y = \dfrac{1}{3}(x - 4)$

3) $y = x$

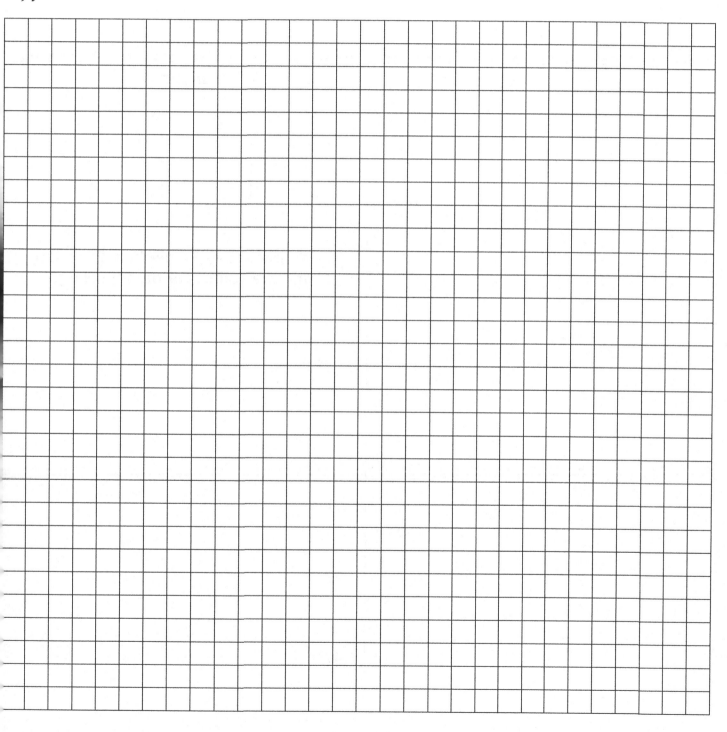

PIECE-WISE FUNCTIONS

What is a Piece-Wise Function:	**Example:**
	$$f(x) = \begin{cases} x+2 & \text{when } x < -1 \\ -x^2 & \text{when } -1 \leq x \leq 3 \\ \frac{3}{4}x+7 & \text{when } x > 3 \end{cases}$$
How do you graph a Piece-Wise Function:	**How do you find the value of a Piece-Wise Function:** $$f(x) = \begin{cases} x+2 & \text{when } x < -1 \\ -x^2 & \text{when } -1 \leq x \leq 3 \\ \frac{3}{4}x+7 & \text{when } x > 3 \end{cases}$$ **Using the above Piece-Wise Function, find the values for the following:** $f(-5) =$ $f(0) =$ $f(4) =$

74

GRAPH OF A PIECE-WISE FUNCTION

Graph the following Piece-Wise Function:

$$y = \begin{cases} x+2 & \text{when} \quad x < -1 \\ -x^2 & \text{when} \quad -1 \leq x \leq 3 \\ \dfrac{3}{4}x + 7 & \text{when} \quad x > 3 \end{cases}$$

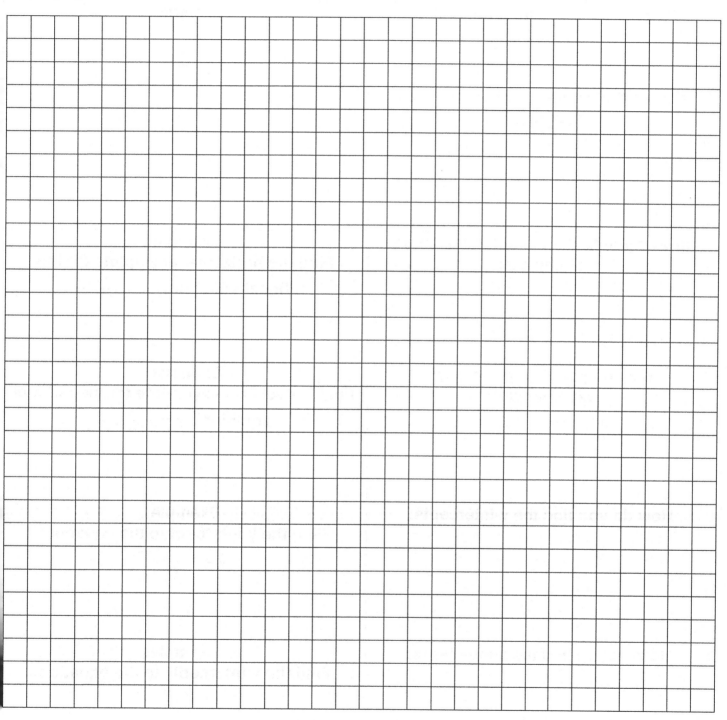

RATIONAL FUNCTIONS

What is a Rational Equation, and what shape is its graph:	Example: $$y = \frac{2x^2 + 3x - 5}{x^2 - 4}$$
What is the basic Absolute Value Equation: **What do the values of a, h, and k do to the graph:** a: h: k:	Example: $$y = \frac{1}{(x-1)} + 5$$
How do you find the find the horizontal asymptote:	Example: Find the horizontal asymptote for the rational equation: $y = \frac{2x^2+3x-5}{x^2-4}$
How do you find the vertical asymptote(s):	Example: Find the vertical asymptote for the rational equation: $y = \frac{2x^2+3x-5}{x^2-4}$
How do you find the y-intercepts:	Example: Find the y-intercept to the equation: $y = \frac{2x^2+3x-5}{x^2-4}$
How do you find the x-intercepts:	Example: Find the x-intercepts to the equation: $y = \frac{2x^2+3x-5}{x^2-4}$

GRAPHS OF RATIONAL FUNCTIONS

Graph the following equation:

1) $y = (2x^2 + 3x - 5)/(x^2 - 4)$

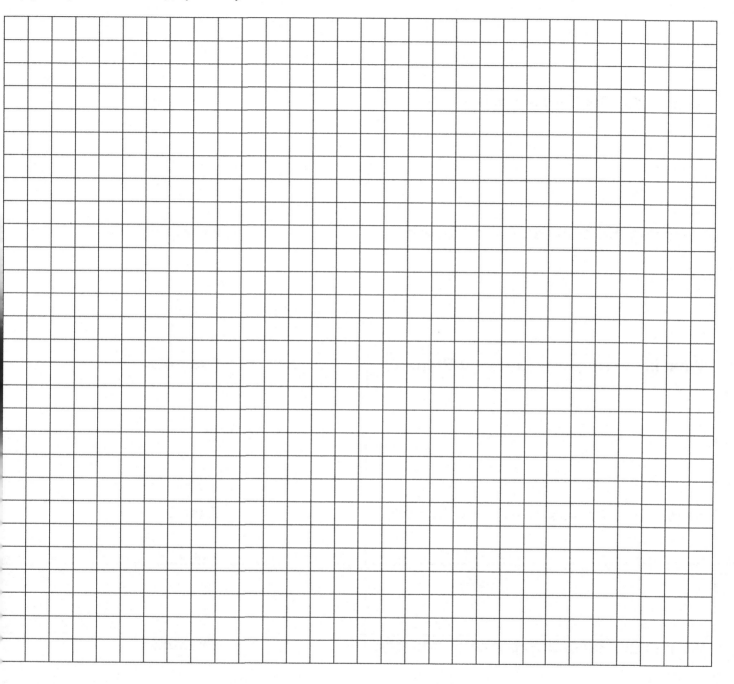

PROPERTIES OF EXPONENTS

What is the Product of Powers Property:	**Example:** $x^3 \cdot x^7 =$
What is the Quotient of Powers Property:	**Example:** $\dfrac{x^7}{x^3} =$ $\dfrac{x^3}{x^7} =$
What is the Zero Exponent Property:	**Example:** $x^0 =$
What is the Negative Exponent Property:	**Example:** $\dfrac{1}{x^3} =$ $x^{-5} =$
What is the Powers of a Power Property:	**Example:** $(x^3)^6 =$
What is the Rational Exponents Property:	**Example:** $x^{\frac{3}{4}} =$ $\sqrt[3]{x^5} =$

EXPONENTIAL EQUATIONS

What is an Exponential Equation, and what shape is its graph: What do the values of a, h, and k do to the graph: a: h: k:	Example: $f(x) = 2^{x-3} + 7$
Where is the horizontal asymptote for an Exponential Equation:	Example: $f(x) = 2^{x-3} + 7$
Where is the y-intercept for an Exponential Equation:	Example: $f(x) = 2^{x-3} + 7$
How do you solve Exponential Equations:	Example: $f(x) = 2^{x-3} + 7$
What is Domain? What is Range:	What is the relationship between Exponential Equations and Logarithms?

GRAPHS OF EXPONENTIAL EQUATIONS

Graph the following equations on the same axis to see what happens:

1) $y = 2^x$

2) $y = \left(\dfrac{1}{2}\right)^x$

3) $y = 2^x + 4$

4) $y = 2^{x-1} + 4$

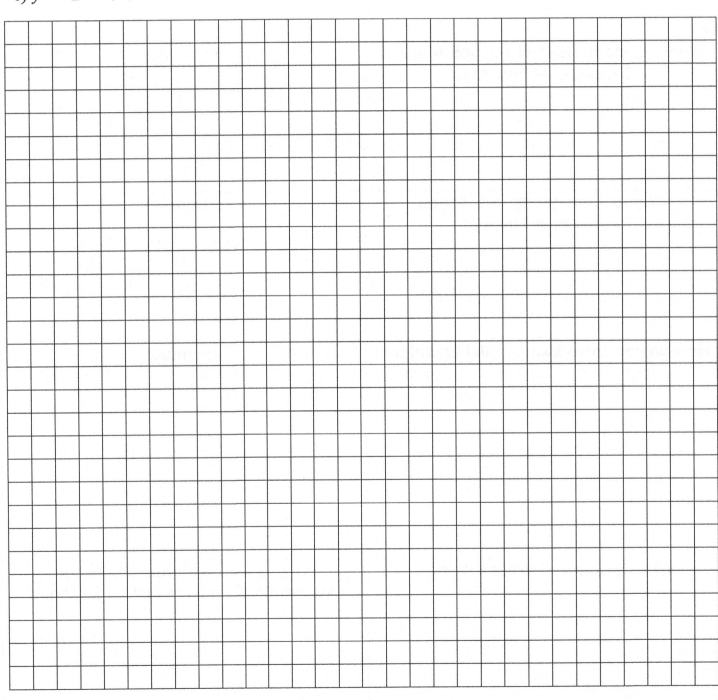

PROPERTIES OF LOGARITHMS

What is a Common Log:	**Example:** $\log 100 =$
What is a Natural Log:	**Example:** $\ln e =$
What is the Multiplication Property of Logs:	**Example:** $\log(8 \cdot 7) =$
What is the Division Property of Logs:	**Example:** $\log\left(\dfrac{56}{7}\right) =$
What is the Powers Property of Logs:	**Example:** $\log(5^2) =$
What is the Change of Base Property of Logs:	**Example:** $\log_9 81 =$

EXTRAS YOU SHOULD KNOW:

1) $\log_b 1 =$

2) $\log_b b =$

3) $\log_b b^2 =$

4) $\log_a b =$

5) $\log_b b^x =$

6) $b^{\log_b x} =$

LOGARITHMIC EQUATIONS

What is a Logarithmic Equation: **What do the values of a, h, and k do to the graph:** a: h: k:	**Example:** $y = \log_2 x$
Where is the vertical asymptote for a Logarithmic Equation:	**Example:** $y = \log_2 x$
Where is the x-intercept for a Logarithmic Equation:	**Example:** $y = \log_2 x$
How do you solve a Logarithmic Equation:	**Example:** $10 = 4 + \log_3(7x)$
What is the relationship between Exponential Equations and Logarithms:	Change the following logarithmic equation into an exponential equation: $y = \log_2 x$ Change the following exponential equation into a logarithmic equation: $2^x = y$

GRAPHS OF LOGARITHMIC EQUATIONS

Graph the following equations on the same axis to see what happens:

1) $y = \log_2 x$

2) $y = \log_2(x + 5)$

3) $y = 3 + \log_2(x + 5)$

4) $y = 3 - \log_2(x + 5)$

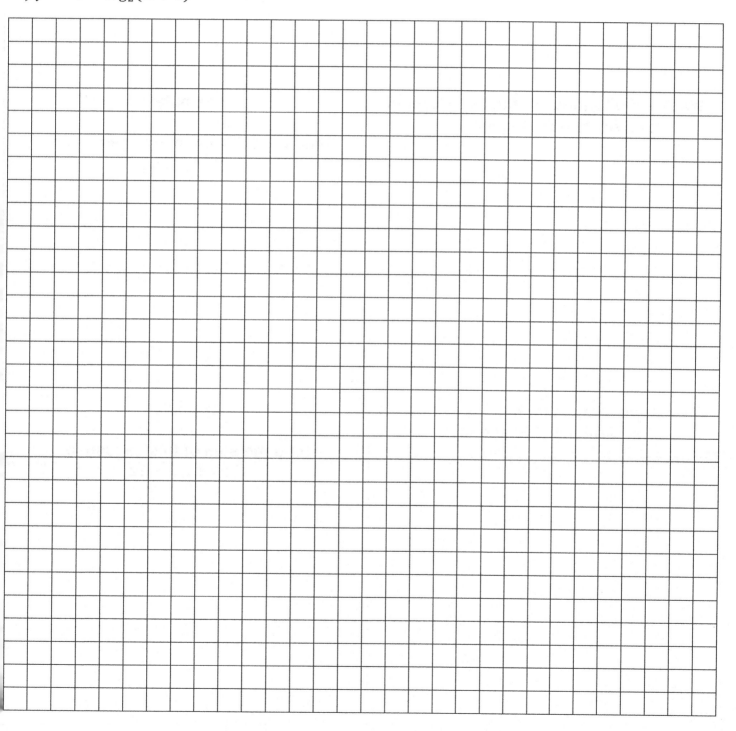

ARITHMETIC SEQUENCES

What is an Arithmetic Sequence:	**Example:** −3,1,5,9,13 ...
What is a Common Difference:	**Example:** −3,1,5,9,13 ... Common difference=
What is the formula for finding a term in an Arithmetic Sequence:	**Example:** **Find the 11th term in this sequence:** −3,1,5,9,13 ...
What is the formula for finding the sum of an Arithmetic Sequence:	**Example:** **Find the sum of this sequence:** 11,7,4,1, ... − 12

GEOMETRIC SEQUENCES

What is a Geometric Sequence:	Example: $$27, 9, 3, \frac{1}{3}, \frac{1}{9} \ldots$$
What is a Common Ratio:	Example: $$27, 9, 3, \frac{1}{3}, \frac{1}{9} \ldots$$ Common Ratio =
What is the formula for finding a term in a Geometric Sequence:	Example: Find the 7th term in this sequence: $$27, 9, 3, \frac{1}{3}, \frac{1}{9} \ldots$$
What is the formula for finding the sum of a Geometric Sequence:	Example: Find the sum of this sequence: $$27, 9, 3, \frac{1}{3}, \frac{1}{9} \ldots$$
What is the Compound Interest Formula:	Example: A man invests $10,000 in an account that pays 8.5% interest per year, compounded quarterly. What is the amount of money that he will have after 3 years?

COMBINATIONS AND PERMUTATIONS

What is a Combination:	**What is a Permutation:**
What is the formula for a Combination when repetition is allowed:	**What is the formula for a Permutation when repetition is allowed:**
What is the formula for a Combination when repetition is <u>not</u> allowed:	**What is the formula for a Permutation when repetition is <u>not</u> allowed:**
What is a factoral:	**What is Pascal's Triangle and how does it help with Permutations:**
Example: If a coach must choose 5 starters from a team of 12 players. How many different potential "starter" teams could he have?	**Example:** If you must pick a number for your locker at school and your lock is three digits long, how many different lock combinations can you have? (Be careful with the misuse of the word "combination")

BASICS OF STATISTICS

What is a Mean/Average? How do you find it:	**Example:** Find the Mean of the following list of numbers: 2,2,3,5,7,13,19,25
What is a Median? How do you find it:	**Example:** Find the Median of the following list of numbers: 2,2,3,5,7,13,19,25
What is a Mode? How do you find it:	**Example:** Find the Mode of the following list of numbers: 2,2,3,5,7,13,19,25
What is a Histrogram: What is a Bar Graph:	**What is a Scatter Plot:**
What is a Box and Whisker graph: **What is the Lower Extreme:** **What is Quartile 1:** **What is the Median:** **What is Quartile 3:** **What is the Upper Extreme:**	**Example:** Create a Box and Whisker Graph with the following set of numbers: 2,2,3,5,7,13,19,25
What is a Bell Curve with a Normal Distribution?	**What is a Standard Deviation?**
What is a Z-score?	**What is the connection between a Z-score and the percent of data on the Bell Curve?**

BASICS OF TRIGONOMETRY

Use the following Unit Circle to label both Degrees and Radians:

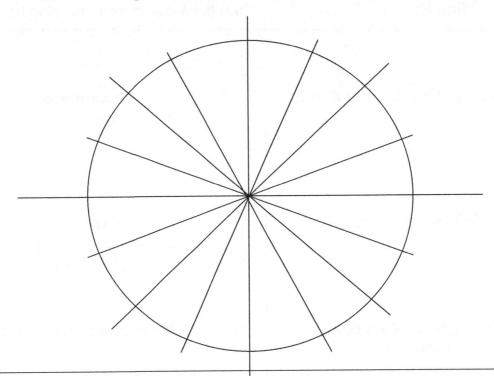

List the ratios for the following:		
Sin θ =	Cos θ =	Tan θ =
Csc θ =	Sec θ =	Cot θ =

Label the Special Right Triangles:

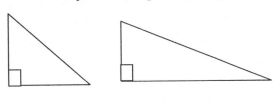

How do you convert from Degrees to Radians:

How do you convert from Radians to Degrees:

Complete the following Table of Values:

Degrees	0°	30°	45°	60°	90°	120°	135°	150°	180°	210°	225°	240°	270°	300°	315°	330°	360°
Radians																	
Sin θ																	
Cos θ																	
Tan θ																	

TRIGONOMETRIC GRAPHS

Basic Sine Function   **Notes about the graph:**

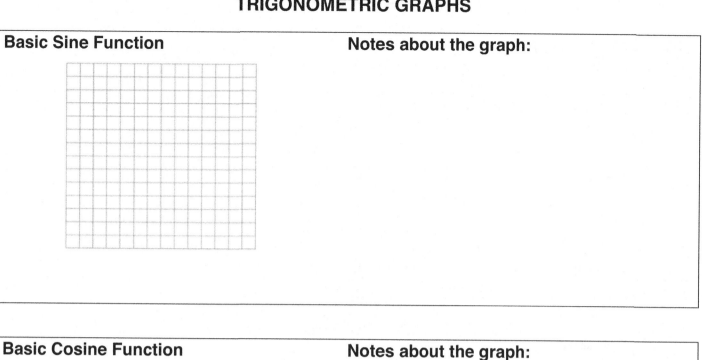

Basic Cosine Function   **Notes about the graph:**

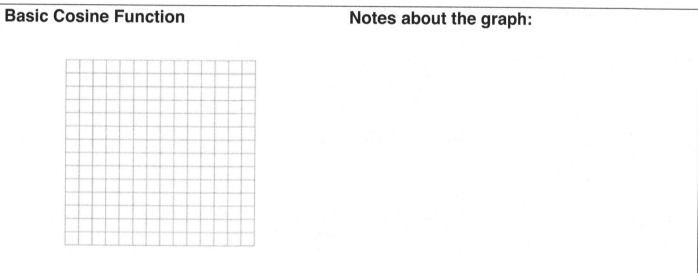

Basic Tangent Function   **Notes about the graph:**

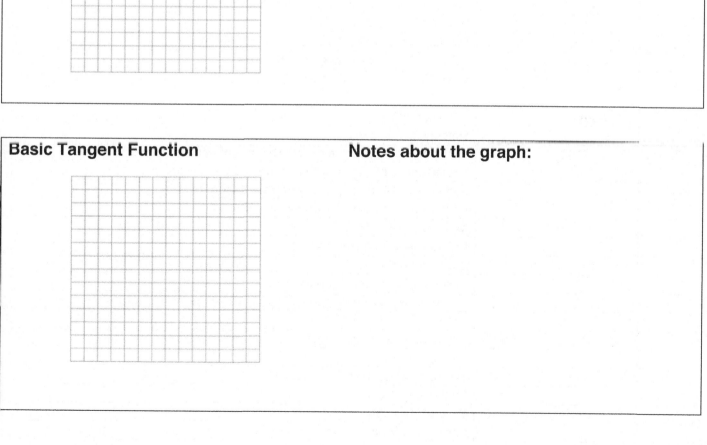

MATH MASTERY CHECKLIST

☑	Math Concepts	Mastery List
	Number Sense	Counting to 100
		Counting by 2's
		Counting by 5's
		Counting by 10's
		Place Value
	Addition	One digit by one digit
		Multiple digits
		Carrying
		Story Problems / Application
	Subtraction	One digit by one digit
		Multiple digits
		Borrowing
		Story Problem / Application
	Multiplication	
		Through 10's
		Through 12's
		One digit by multiple digit
		Multiple digit by multiple digit
		Story Problems / Application
	Division	Short division through 12's
		Long division with one digit divisor
		Long division with one digit divisor and remainders
		Long with 2+ digit divisors
		Division – long with 2+ digit divisors and remainders
		Rules of Divisibility (2's, 3's, 5's, 9's, 10's)
		Story Problems / Application
	Fractions	Naming Fractions
		Simplifying Fractions
		Changing Fractions from proper to improper and improper to proper
		Adding and subtracting with common denominators
		Adding and subtracting with different denominators
		Adding and subtracting with mixed numbers
		Multiplying fractions
		Multiplying with mixed numbers
		Dividing fractions
		Dividing with mixed numbers
		Story Problems / Application
	Decimals	Converting fractions to decimals
		Adding decimals
		Subtracting decimals
		Multiplying decimals
		Dividing decimals
		Conversion from a decimal to a percent

			Conversion from a fraction to a decimal to a percent
			Story Problems / Application
		Integers	Adding integers
			Subtracting integers
			Multiplying integers
			Dividing integers
			Order of Operations (PEMDAS)
			Properties of Numbers – Commutative, Associative, Distributive, Identity, etc.
			Story Problems / Application
		Algebraic Terms	Adding Algebraic Terms
			Subtracting Algebraic Terms
			Multiplying Algebraic Terms
			Dividing Algebraic Terms
		Equations	Solving for one variable – addition property
			Solving for one variable – subtraction property
			Solving for one variable – multiplication property
			Solving for one variable – division property
			Multi-step Equations
			Work Equations
			Distance/Rate/Time Equations
			Mixture Equations
		Polynomials	Adding polynomials
			Subtracting polynomials
			Multiplying a monomial by a polynomial (Distributive Property)
			Multiplying a binomial by a binomial (FOIL)
			Multiplying polynomials by polynomials
			Dividing polynomials by factoring - factoring trinomials without an "a" term - factoring trinomials with an "a" term - factoring by grouping
			Dividing polynomials by long division
			Dividing polynomials by synthetic division
		Rational Equations	Multiplying rational polynomials
			Dividing rational polynomials
			Adding and Subtracting rational polynomials with common denominators
			Adding and Subtracting rational polygons without common denominators
			Solving rational equations
		Graphing	Cartesian Plans – plotting points
		Linear Equations	Definition of a linear equation
			Patterns of growth in number sequences/tiles
			Graphing tables of values
			Identifying slope and y-intercepts
			Writing linear equations in slope-intercept form $y = mx + b$
			Graphing linear equations in slope-intercept form $y = mx + b$
			Slope formula - Finding slope given two points

		Graphing linear equations in standard form ax + by = c
		Graphing linear equations in point-slope form $y-y_1 = m(x-x_1)$
		Writing linear equations given a slope and y-intercept
		Writing linear equations given a point and slope
		Writing linear equations given two points
	Linear Inequalities	Solving inequalities – addition and subtraction property
		Solving inequalities – multiplication and division property
		Graphing inequalities on a number line (open/closed dots and shading)
		Graphing linear inequalities on a Cartesian Plane (dotted lines, solid lines and shading)
	Systems of Equations	Solve by graphing
		Solve by substitution
		Solve by elimination
	Quadratic Equations	Definition of a quadratic equation
		The basic shape of the graph of a quadratic equation
		Forms of the quadratic equation: Standard form
		Forms of the quadratic equation: Vertex form - Knowledge of how "a" transforms the graph - Knowledge of how "h" transforms the graph - Knowledge of how "k" transforms the graph
		Finding the y-intercept with both equations
		Finding the x-intercept/zeros of the equation - Factoring - Completing the Square - Quadratic Equation
		Finding the vertex - (h, k) - $(-\frac{b}{2a}, f(x))$ - Changing an equation from standard form to vertex form by completing the square
	Exponents	Scientific Notation - With positive Exponents - With negative Exponents
		Simplifying exponents using properties of exponents - Zero Property - Product of Powers Property - Quotient of Powers Property - Negative Exponents Property - Power of a Power Property
	Functions	Functions vs. Relations
		Domain and Range
	Cubic Function	Basic Graph - Knowledge of how "a" transforms the graph - Knowledge of how "h" transforms the graph - Knowledge of how "k" transforms the graph

	Inverse Functions	How to find an Inverse function
		The relationship between a function and its inverse
		Graphs of a function and its inverse
		How to find the domain and range
	Piece-Wise Functions	How to graph a Piece-Wise function
		How to find an f(x) value given an x value
		How to find the domain and range
	Polynomial Functions	How to determine the number of zeros
		How to find the zeros - Long division - Synthetic division
		End behavior and sign charts
		Graphing Polynomial Functions
	Sequences	Arithmetic Sequences
		Geometric Sequences
		Permutations and Combinations
	Statistics	Mean
		Median
		Mode
		Range and Midrange
		Histographs, Bar Graphs, Scatterplots
		Box and Whisker Plots: 5 Number Summary
		Bell Curve
		Standard Deviation
		Z-Scores
	Trigonometry	Unit Circle
		Trigonometric Ratios
		Special Right Triangles
		Converting Radians to Degrees and Degrees to Radians
		Table of Values
		Graphs of Sine, Cosine and Tangent